Pooja's SOULFUL RECIPES

TOP SMOOTHIE RECIPES

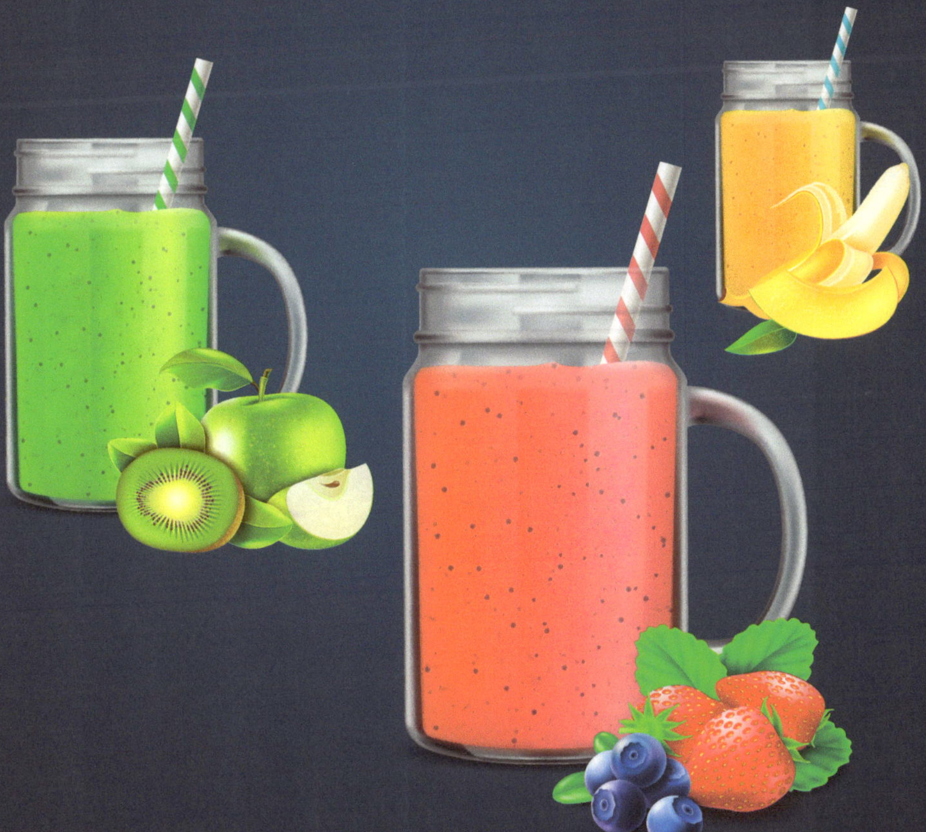

DISCOVER THE TEN MOST DELICIOUS AND NUTRITIOUS SMOOTHIE RECIPES

BOOK INTRODUCTION

Top Healthy Smoothies is an inspiring and informative book of poojas soulful recipes. It is a collection of easy-to-follow healthy smoothie recipes that are both delicious and nutritious. This book is full of ideas for quick, healthy smoothies that can be enjoyed by everyone.

It includes an array of smoothie combinations, from simple fruit and vegetable smoothies to more complex and flavourful smoothies. The book contains all the information needed to make these smoothies, including how to select and prepare the ingredients, how to blend them together, and how to make them taste great. It also includes tips and tricks to make the perfect smoothie and ideas for different ways to enjoy them. For those looking to make a healthier lifestyle change, this book is a great resource. With Poojas Soulful recipes, Top Healthy Smoothies will help you create delicious and nutritious smoothies that you and your family can enjoy.

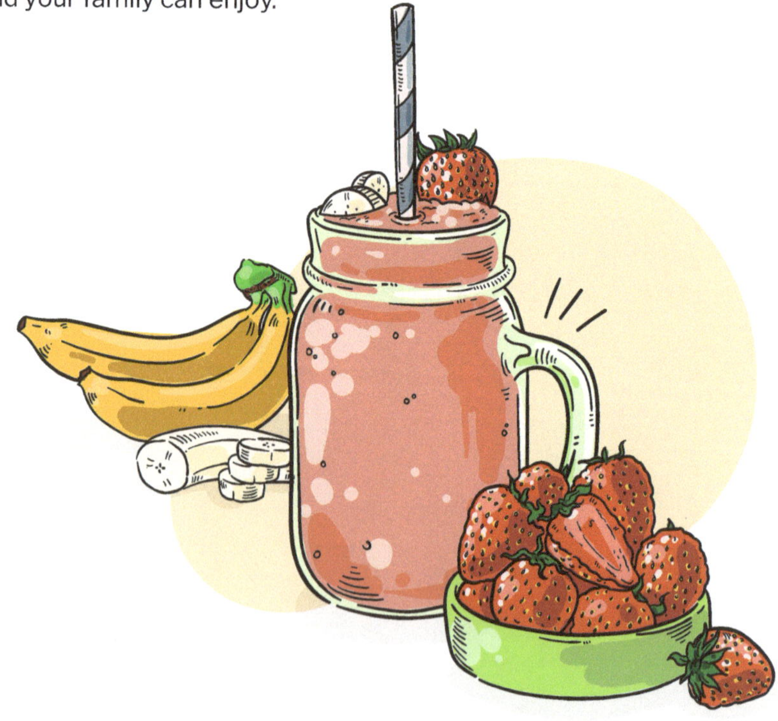

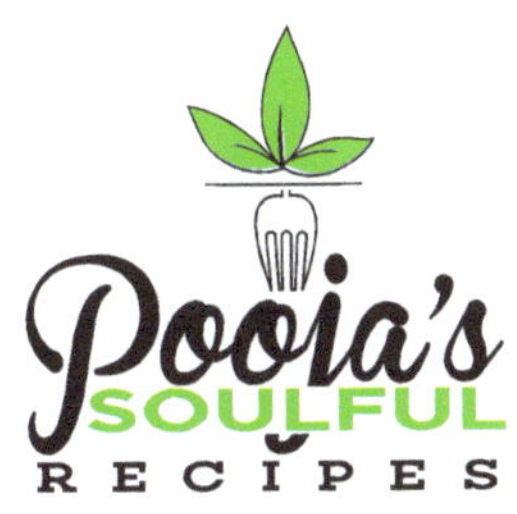

Hi,

I am Pooja Patil. I have done my Computer Engineering and helping thousands of Doctors to build their clinical practice through digital marketing and helping heart, diabetes, hypertension and obesity patients to reach right point of care so that they can conquer their disease.

But one thing I want to tell you is I am very much passionate about cooking. Cooking Comes from my soul and that's why the name 'Pooja's Soulful recipes' So far I have created hundreds of videos of healthy recipes for the brand 'Madhavbaug' for their MibPulse Application, YouTube, Facebook and Instagram which we have developed to help the heart patients regarding their diet at home .

One thing I must tell you that I had never explored cooking before marriage because I never really had the time, but after marriage, I found myself some time to indulge in trial and error to improve my cooking skills.

I am a passionate foodie with a profound enthusiasm for flavorful and nutritious meals. My purpose in life is to share my cooking expertise and passion for food with the world. Over the past 10 years, I have been honing my culinary skills and creating inventive recipes for my blog. I strongly believe that it is essential to eat healthily and nutritiously and I enjoy experimenting with different ingredients and flavors. My first book, Top Smoothie Recipes, is filled with a variety of smoothie recipes that will tantalize your taste buds. From traditional recipes to unconventional and exciting flavors, you are certain to find a recipe that you will love! Whether you are looking for a scrumptious breakfast or snack, or something to cool you off on a hot summer day, my book is sure to have the perfect solution.

AUTHOR TESTIMONIAL

Dr. Rohit Sane, CEO and MD Madhavbaug

I know Pooja from last few years. In Covid time she has helped many of my patients with her healthy and tasty recipes to manage their disease. She is passionate about her cooking and with her book now she can help many such patients to cook healthy and tasty recipes. I wish her all the very best.

Dr. Deepali Amin, MD, Care Partners Madhavbaug

I have attended Pooja's healthy salads workshop. My patients learnt so much about variety of salads and I am sure that it will help them to build positive eating habits and help them to reverse their chronic diseases such as diabetes, high blood pressure, obesity, and heart. I wish Pooja all the very best for this book and future endeavours.

Dr. Harsha Mahajan, Care Partner Madhavbaug

This book is a collection of the 10 best smoothies which is a perfect formula to shed some extra kilos. Pooja has done awesome work and I am sure that she will create many more to help my patients to reverse their disease.

Madhura Walawalkar, Professional Singer

I am professional singer but I was struggling with the health issues. I was suffering from acid reflux and weight issues. With Pooja's magical healthy and tasty food recipes I was able to fight with these diseases successfully. I feel that her mantra of food is our medicine has worked for me very well and I am sure it will work for many others with this book. I wish her all the very best for this book and I am sure that with her skills she can write many more.

DEDICATION

This book is dedicated to all the heart, diabetics, hypertension, obese patients who would like to create the smoothies mentioned in the book. To lose weight and reverse their disease.

TABLE OF CONTENTS

APPLE OAT SMOOTHIE

This Apple Oat Smoothie is a great way to start the day! Fruity, nutty, and with a sprinkle of cinnamon, this healthy oat-filled beverage is the perfect breakfast in a cup.

Prep Time: 5 mins

Calories: 329kcal

Author: Pooja

Ingredients

- 1 medium apple, peeled and cored
- 1/4 cup rolled oats
- 1 tbsp. almond butter or other nut butter
- 1/4 tsp. cinnamon
- /2 cup oat milk

Instructions

1. First, core and slice your apple. You might want to remove the skin, but that's up to you. Then, add all of the ingredients to a blender and cover it with the lid.

2. Process the smoothie on high until the chunks of fruit are gone and it's smooth. Pour it into a glass and enjoy promptly.

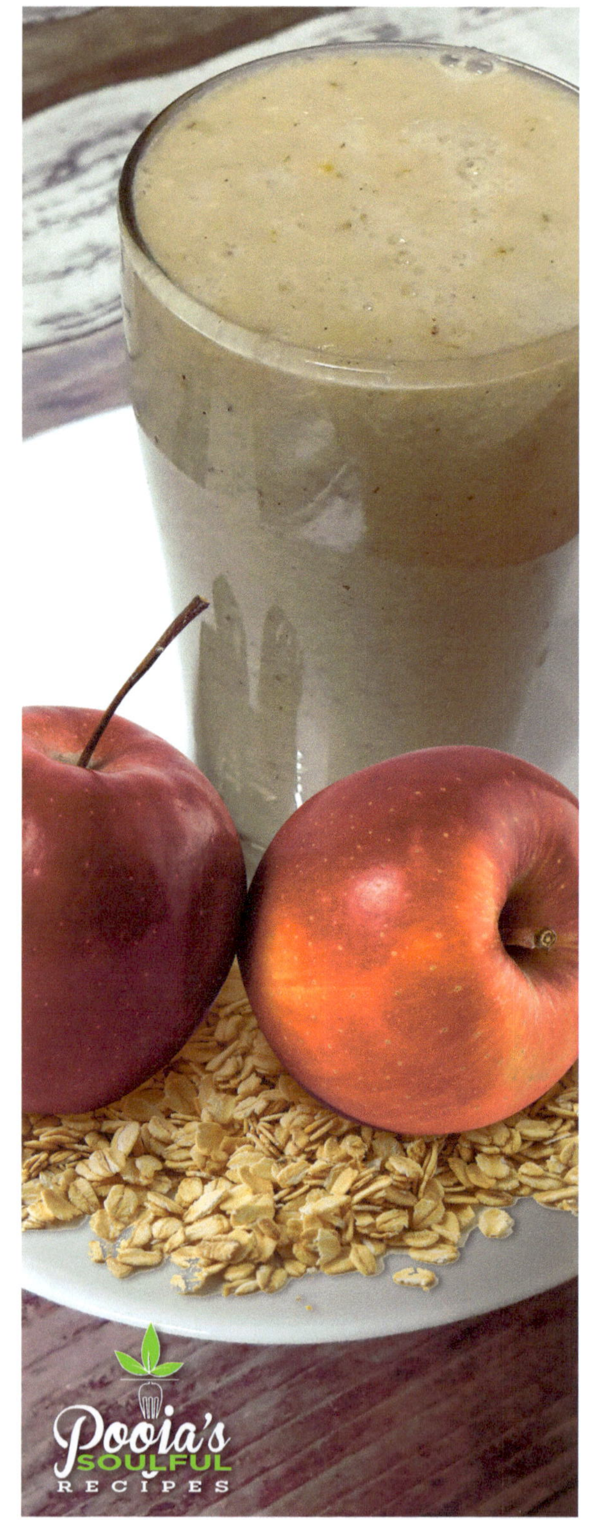

HOW TO MAKE THE BEST SMOOTHIE

• Choose the right apple. To get that smooth texture and sweet flavor, make sure that you choose an apple that is not over-ripe or mealy. You want to get one that is firm to the touch and doesn't give when you press lightly on the skin.

• Keep your ingredients cold. Smoothies taste best cold, so try to keep your ingredients cold as well or the results will be lukewarm. Except for the oats and cinnamon, I suggest storing the rest in the fridge for a chilled morning drink. You may also add a few ice cubes, of course.

• Stir if needed. If you find you're getting chunks in your Apple Oat Smoothie, use the attachment or a spoon (when the blender is off or unplugged) to stir the ingredients so everything blends smoothly and incorporates together. Nut butter can sometimes get stuck to the walls of the blender and needs to be dislodged.

Nutrition

Calories: 329kcal | Carbohydrates: 54g | Protein: 8g | Fat: 11g | Saturated Fat: 1g | Sodium: 61mg | Potassium: 443mg | Fiber: 10g | Sugar: 29g | Vitamin A: 348IU | Vitamin C: 8mg | Calcium: 258mg | Iron: 3mg

DELICIOUS DATE SMOOTHIE

Time	: Max 10 Min
Calories	: 150-450 Kcal
Diet	: Dairy-free, Egg- Free, Gluten-free, Vegan
Prep Time	: 3 Minutes
Servings	: 1 Person
Calories	: 403 Kcal

INGREDIENTS
- 1 banana (ideally frozen the night before)
- 1 ¼ cups oat milk (or your fav plant-based milk)
- 4 dates, dried
- 1 tbsp flax seeds
- 1 tsp cinnamon

INSTRUCTIONS
1. Making sure your banana is peeled, throw it into your smoothie maker/food processor.

2. Add the milk, dates, flax seeds and cinnamon. Give it a good blend.

3. Done! Easy peasy.

NUTRITION
Calories: 403kcal | Carbohydrates: 82g | Protein: 8g | Fat: 7g | Sodium: 146mg | Potassium: 835mg | Fiber: 11g | Sugar: 55g | Vitamin A: 690IU | Vitamin C: 10.2mg | Calcium: 494mg | Iron: 3.6mg

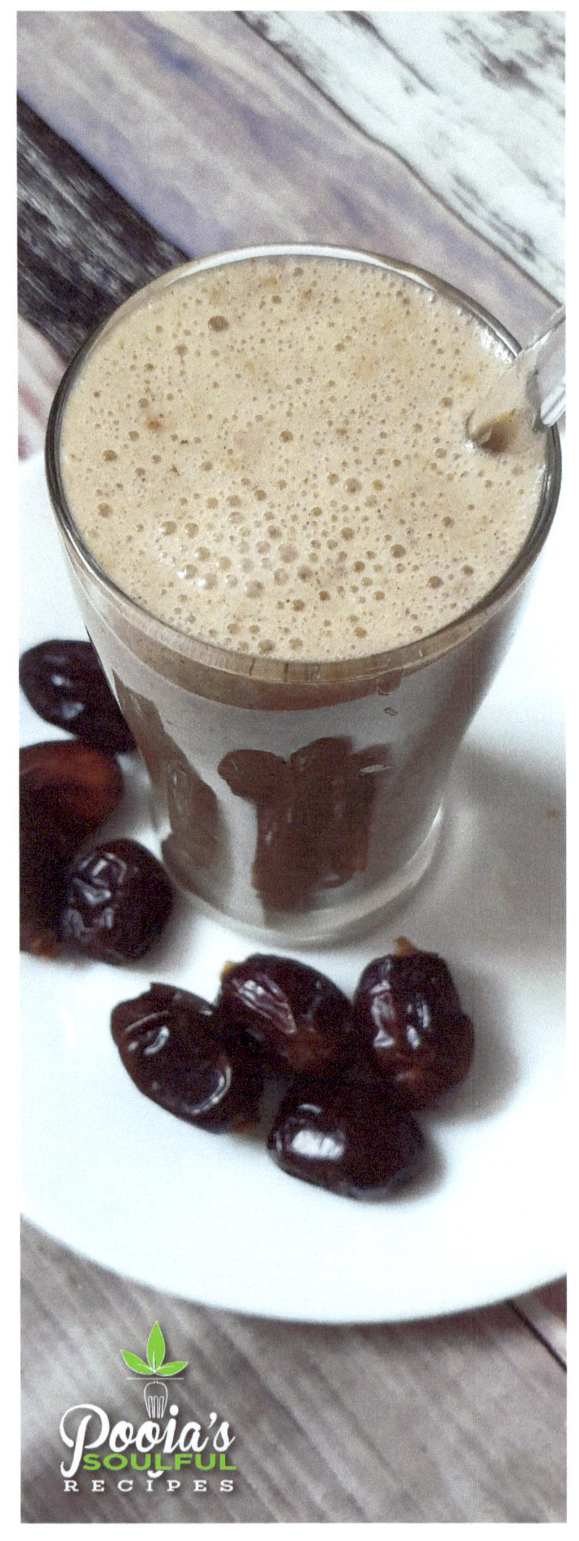

STRAWBERRY PINEAPPLE SMOOTHIE

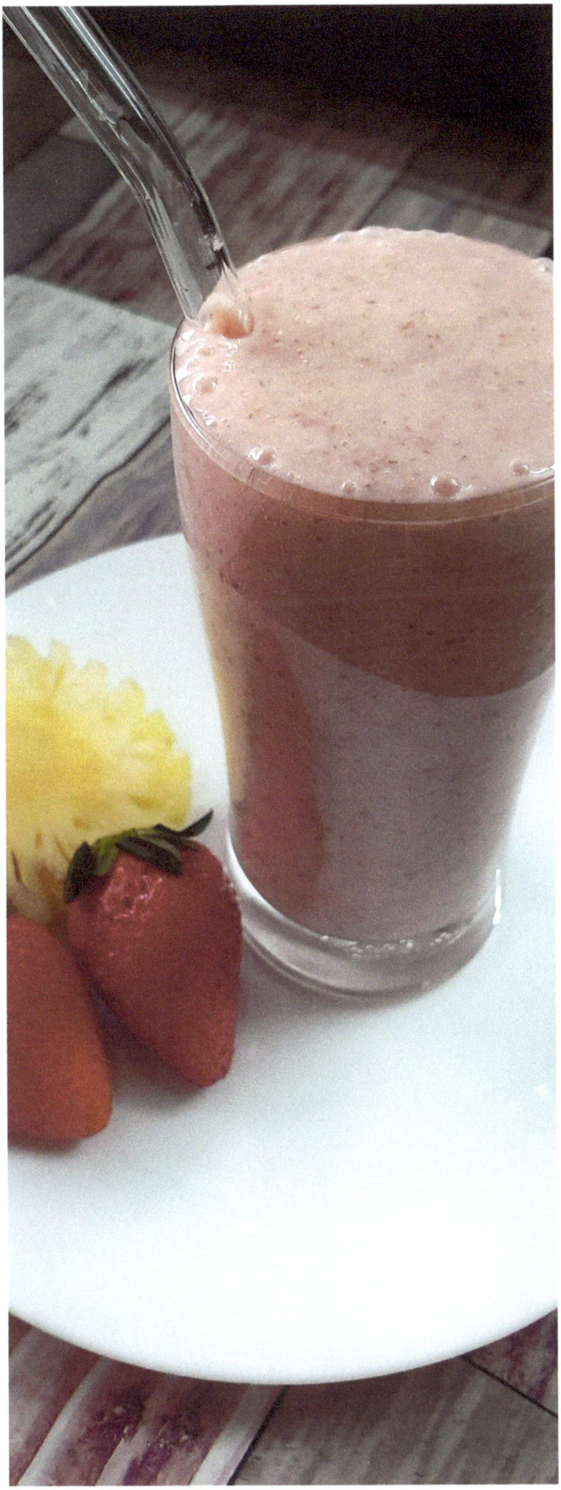

Enjoy tropical flavours combined with a healthy dose of protein in this mouthwatering strawberry pineapple smoothie.

Prep Time : 5 mins

Servings : 1 Serving

Calories : 256kcal

INGREDIENTS :

- 5-6 strawberries fresh or frozen
- 1/3 cup pineapple fresh or frozen
- 1 ripe banana
- 1 tablespoon hemp hearts
- 1/2 cup almond milk or milk of choice a little more as needed if using frozen fruit

INSTRUCTIONS :

1. Add all the ingredients to your blender and process until smooth. Enjoy!

Pooja's SOULFUL RECIPES

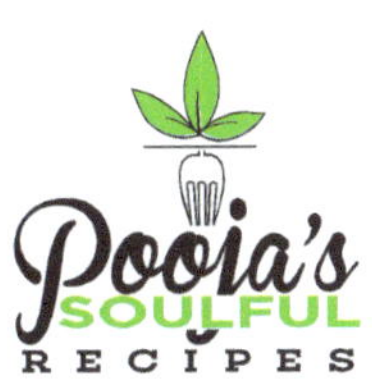

Notes -

Depending on the ratio of fresh or frozen fruit, **you may need to adjust the liquid quantity.** Fresh fruit is easier to blend and naturally has more liquid, so use only half a cup of plant milk with all fresh fruit. Add more milk as needed when using frozen fruit.

Frozen fruit will give thicker, creamier results, but fresh fruit also works well, as the banana will slightly thicken your strawberry pineapple smoothie.

For extra slush and to thicken your drink when using fresh fruit, add a handful of ice cubes. Skip when using frozen fruit.

If you do not have hemp hearts, you may sub for a tablespoon of flax seeds, ground flax, chia seeds, or even a nut butter such as almond or peanut butter.

For extra sweetness, add 1-2 pitted dates or a teaspoon of maple or date syrup. I find this smoothie to be plenty sweet as is, but if you like it extra sweet, make it to your liking.

If you don't have pineapple, mango also works well as a replacement. Raspberries or cherries also work well to sub the strawberries if you don't have any on hand.

The recipe makes approx 2 cups, enough for one large glass or two smaller servings.

Nutrition

Calories: 256kcal | Carbohydrates: 40g | Protein: 8g | Fat: 8g | Sodium: 164mg | Potassium: 574mg | Fiber: 5g | Sugar: 22g | Vitamin A: 155IU | Vitamin C: 71.9mg | Calcium: 171mg | Iron: 2.6mg

STRAWBERRY BANANA SMOOTHIE

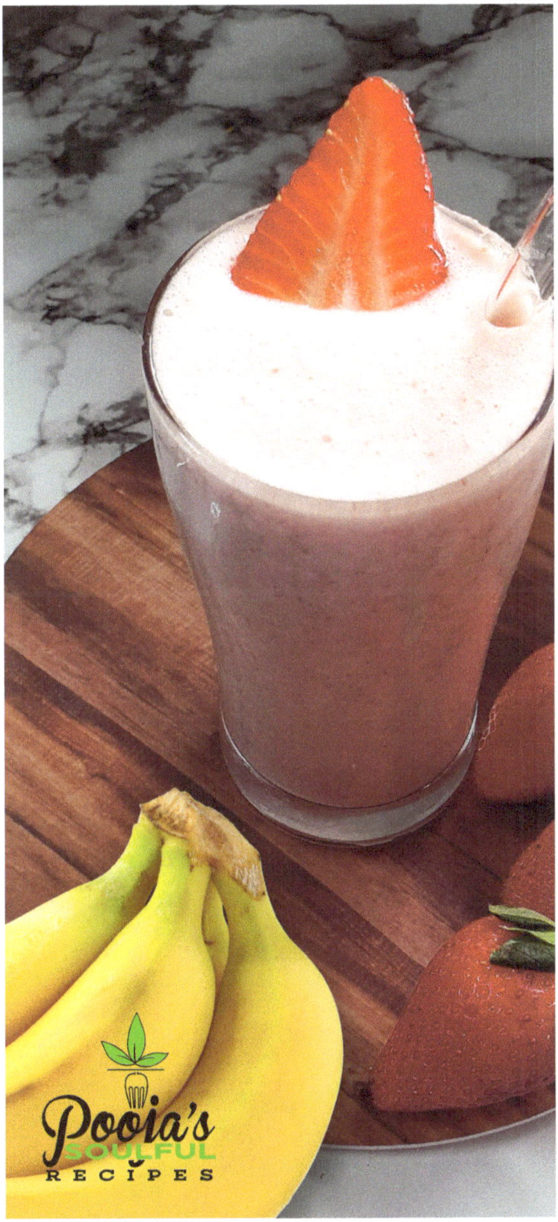

This Strawberry Banana Smoothie is such a treat. It's thick, sweet, and creamy, packed with fruity flavors. It's also filling, low in calories, and has no added sugars.
Perfect healthy breakfast or refreshing energizing drink.

Prep Time : 5 mins
Servings : 1 serving
Calories : 173kcal

EQUIPMENT :
· Blender

INGREDIENTS :
· 1 cup strawberries fresh or frozen
· ½ banana
· 1 cup oat milk
· 1 tablespoon ground flax seeds
· ½ teaspoon Ceylon cinnamon
· Ice cubes
· Sweetener (optional): Maple syrup, honey or dates, to taste

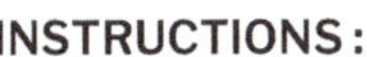

INSTRUCTIONS :
1. Start with preparing and measuring all the ingredients. I like to use measuring cups.
2. If you are using fresh strawberries, wash them and remove strawberry stems.
3. If you have whole flax seeds, make sure you grind them in a grinder before using them.
4. Take the blender and add all ingredients. Note: add wet ingredients first for easier blending.
5. Turn on the blender and mix at high speed until you get a smooth texture.
6. If the smoothie is too thick, add a little more liquid – milk or water. Blend again until the smoothie is smooth.
7. Transfer the smoothie into a tall smoothie glass.
8. Serve and enjoy.

Notes -

As a measure, I used a cup (240ml).

Substitions:

• You can use fresh or frozen fruits.

• You can use any plant-based milk here except coconut milk. Coconut milk (from a box) won't work well here in terms of pairing with other flavors. Cow's milk works well too.

• You can substitute flax seeds with chia seeds or hemp seeds.

This strawberry banana smoothie is **vegan and gluten-free.**

Make it without banana: Substitute banana with ½ avocado. In that case, you will need to add extra sweetener. See the "Sweetener recommendation" for suggestions.

Make it weight loss friendly: Use only ½ banana to cut down calories. Or omit banana and use ¼ avocado. If using avocado, opt-in for low-carb sweeteners, like stevia.

Store in a smoothie cup with a lid and keep refrigerated for up to one day.

***Read the whole recipe post for more tips and information about ingredients and preparation.

NUTRITION :

Serving: 1 serving | Calories: 173kcal | Carbohydrates: 28g | Protein: 4g | Fat: 7g | Saturated Fat: 1g | Sodium: 329mg | Potassium: 488mg | Fiber: 8g | Sugar: 15g | Vitamin C: 89.8mg | Calcium: 341mg | Iron: 1mg

SPINACH BANANA SMOOTHIE

Calories : 150 - 450 Kcal
Prep Time : 3 Minutes
Servings : 1 Big Glass
Calories : 310 Kcal

EQUIPMENT :
• Blender

INGREDIENTS :
• 1 medium banana
• 1 big handful spinach
(1 handful = approx. 60g)
• 1¼ cup unsweetened soy milk (or your fave milk - almond, oat, coconut, even water)

INSTRUCTIONS :
1. Easy as hell - throw everything together!
2. And blend!

NUTRITION :
Serving: 538g | Calories: 310kcal | Carbohydrates: 37g | Protein: 15g | Fat: 13g | Saturated Fat: 2g | Sodium: 226mg | Potassium: 1169mg | Fiber: 6g | Sugar: 17g | Vitamin A: 5395IU | Vitamin C: 24.3mg | Calcium: 426mg | Iron: 3.3mg

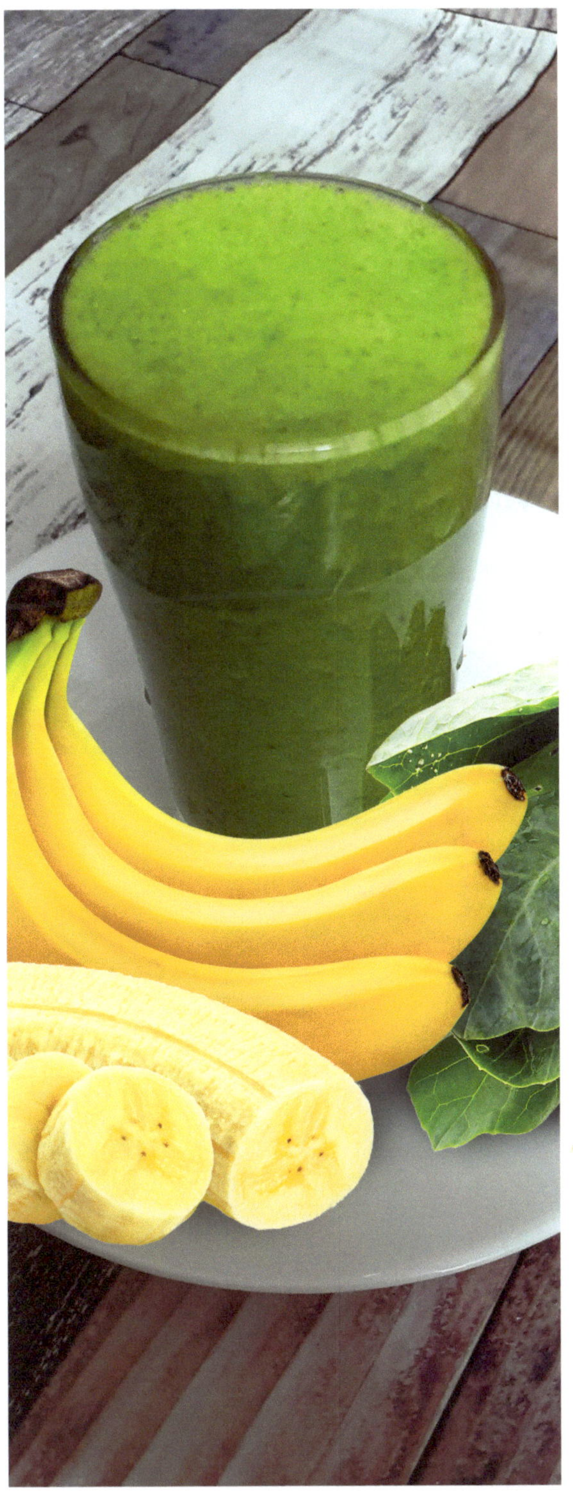

SPICY KIWI BANANA SMOOTHIE

Calories : 150 - 450 Kcal
Prep Time : 3 Minutes
Servings : 2 People
Calories : 297 Kcal

INGREDIENTS

- 3 kiwi
- 2 banana
- ¾ cup milk (any milk is fine, try soy, almond, coconut etc)
- ¾ cup low-fat yogurt
- 4 tbsp porridge oats
- 1 thumb ginger, fresh

OPTIONAL

- 1 tsp honey (if you like it that bit sweeter)

INSTRUCTIONS :

1. Skin the kiwis - chop off the top and bottom, stand and slice off the edges (not your fingers)
2. Peel 2 bananas (a monkey can do it, so can you).
3. Chop or grate the ginger. 1 thumb ginger, fresh.
4. Throw fruits, oats and ginger into a blender with the milk and yoghurt. ¾ cup milk, ¾ cup low-fat yogurt, 1 tsp honey
5. Blend.
6. Drink!

NUTRITION :

Serving: 445g | Calories: 297kcal | Carbohydrates: 59g | Protein: 11g | Fat: 3g | Cholesterol: 3mg | Sodium: 85mg | Potassium: 1106mg | Fiber: 8.9g | Sugar: 28.9g | Vitamin A: 850IU | Vitamin C: 160.1mg | Calcium: 350mg | Iron: 1.6mg

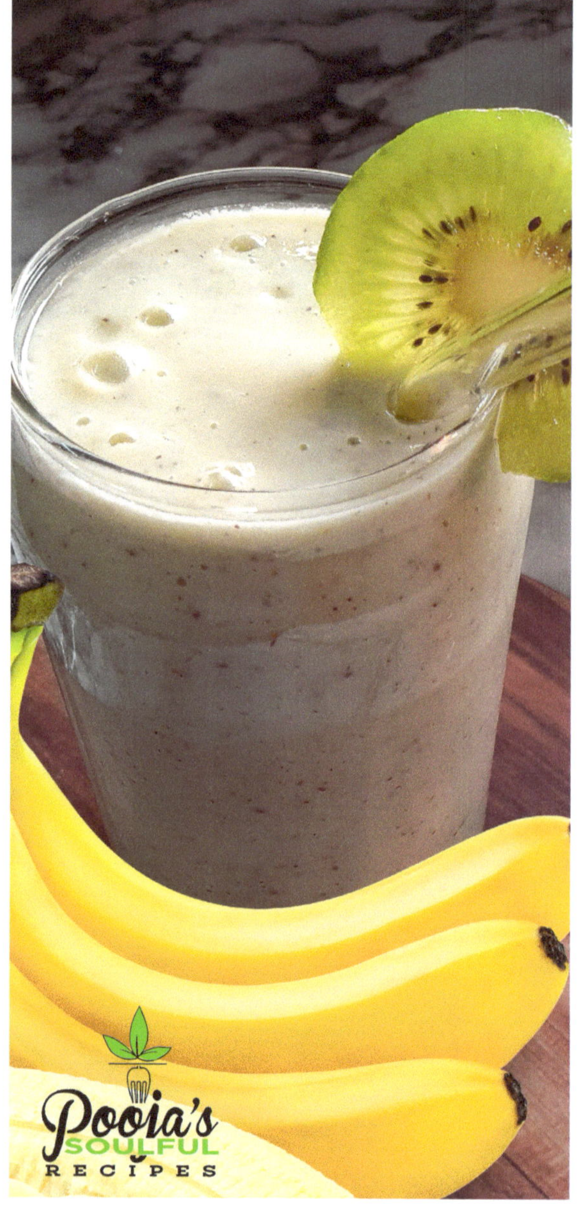

DELICIOUS KALE SMOOTHIE

The only Kale Smoothie Recipe you'll ever need: not only good for you, but also delicious!
This detoxifying protein-packed green smoothie tastes amazingly refreshing and only takes
5 minutes to make!

Prep Time : 2 Minutes
Servings : 2 Servings
Calories : 203 kcal

EQUIPMENT
• Blender, Rubber Spatula
• Culinary Scissors

INGREDIENTS :
• 1 cup or 70 gms Kale
• 1 banana
• 1 tablespoon unsweetened peanut butter
• 1 tablespoon maple syrup or any other sweetener of your choice
• 1 tablespoon lemon juice
• 1 cup or 230 ml unsweetened almond milk or any other nut milk
• Water or ice optional
• A pinch of sea salt

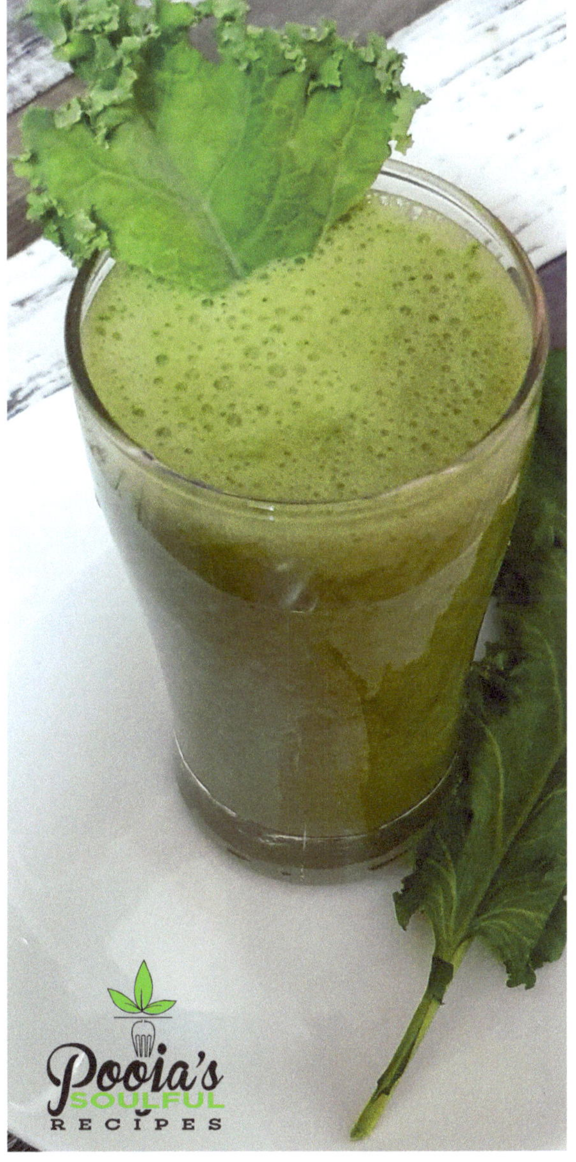

INSTRUCTIONS :
1. Blend all the ingredients in a blender until smooth. Add a bit of ice or water to adjust the consistency and a pinch of salt to balance the taste. Enjoy!

Notes: Top Tips -
• This smoothie will take you no more than 5 minutes to make. Use it as your go-to delicious green smoothie recipe.
• It's better to use ripe bananas. In this case, you will need less sweetener as they are naturally sweeter
• Don't underestimate a pinch of sea salt. It balances the taste of this smoothie making it just right!
• Use water to thin up the smoothie to your liking.
• If you have leftover kale, use it for kale pumpkin salad, vegan casserole with sweet potatoes and kale, harvest salad, buddha bowl or vegan zuppa toscana.

RECIPE VARIATIONS :

• Use any type of Kale for your green smoothie. Most common are curly kale and Tuscan (Lacinato) kale. Here are some more kale varieties that you might want to consider.
• Fresh spinach can be substituted for kale for a delicious green smoothie.
• Use any other sweetener instead of maple syrup: agave juice, date syrup or molasses. You'll need less sweetener if you use ripe bananas.
• Use frozen banana for a creamy chilled effect.
• Any nut milk or oat milk can be substituted for almond milk.

NUTRITION :

Calories : 203kcal | Carbohydrates: 33g | Protein: 8g | Fat: 7g | Saturated Fat: 1g | Sodium: 237mg | Potassium: 874mg | Fiber: 2g | Sugar: 14g | Vitamin A: 11856IU | Vitamin C: 150mg | Calcium: 337mg | Iron: 2mg

BLUEBERRY BANANA PROTEIN SMOOTHIE

Calories : 450 - 650 Kcal
Prep time : 5 Min
Servings : 1 Servings
Calories : 506 Kcal

EQUIPMENT
• Blender
• Grater

INGREDIENTS :
• 1 cup blueberries, frozen
(fresh is fine too)
• 1 ripe banana (make sure
they're soft and sweet!
Keep some in the freezer like
we do here)
• 1 cup milk of choice (we use
soy milk)
• 1 tsp vanilla extract
• 2 tbsp chia seeds
• 1 tsp lemon zest

OPTIONAL
• 1 serving vanilla protein powder (for that extra protein hit!)

INSTRUCTIONS
1. Add all the ingredients to a blender, and grate in the lemon zest.
1 cup blueberries, frozen,1 ripe banana,1 cup milk of choice,1 tsp vanilla extract, 4
oz low fat cottage cheese,2 tbsp chia seeds,1 tsp lemon zest
2. Blend. Done!

NUTRITION :
Calories: 506kcal | Carbohydrates: 71g | Protein: 27g | Fat: 14g | Saturated
Fat: 2g | Polyunsaturated Fat: 9g | Monounsaturated Fat: 2g | Trans Fat: 0.03g |
Cholesterol: 5mg | Sodium: 585mg | Potassium: 1073mg | Fiber: 16g |
Sugar: 39g | Vitamin A: 1143IU | Vitamin C: 45mg | Calcium: 569mg | Iron: 4mg

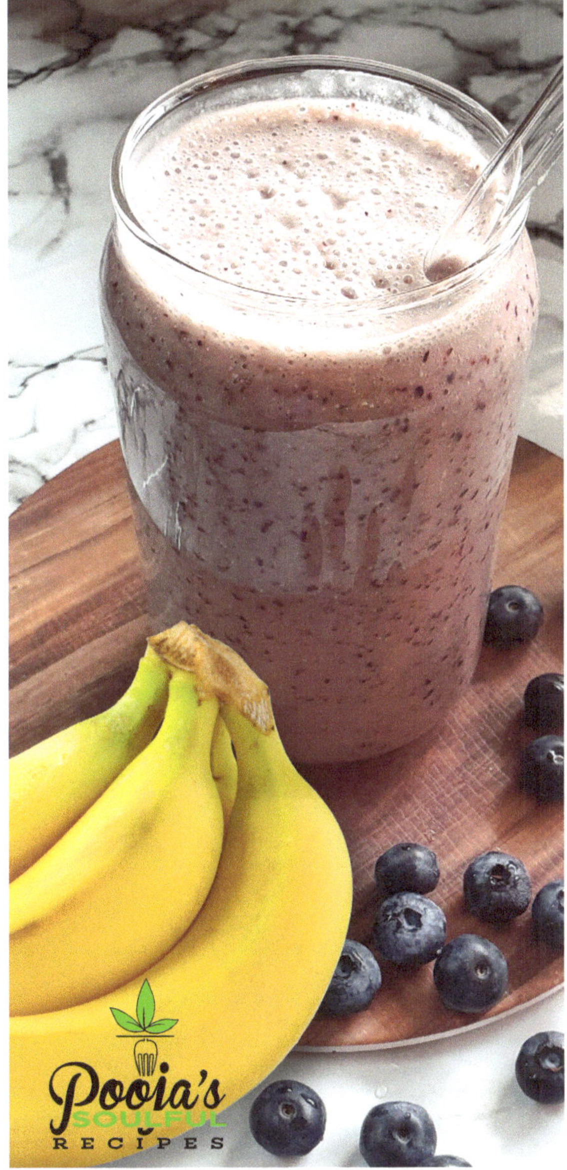

BEET SMOOTHIE

Recipe with Blueberries and Ginger

This vegan beet smoothie recipe is made with raw beets, berries, banana, and ginger. It's sweet, tart, and has a nice earthy flavor and bright pink color from the beets.

Prep Time : 10 minutes

INGREDIENTS :
- 1 small beet, peeled and chopped
- 1 cup frozen blueberries
- 1 inch fresh ginger, peeled
- 1/2 cup frozen banana chunks
- 1 tablespoon sunflower seeds
- 1 cup non-dairy milk
- 1/2 cup water
- Juice of 1/2 lemon

INSTRUCTIONS :
1. Combine all ingredients in a blender and blend until smooth.

2. Add more water or non-dairy milk if you'd like the smoothie to have a thinner consistency.

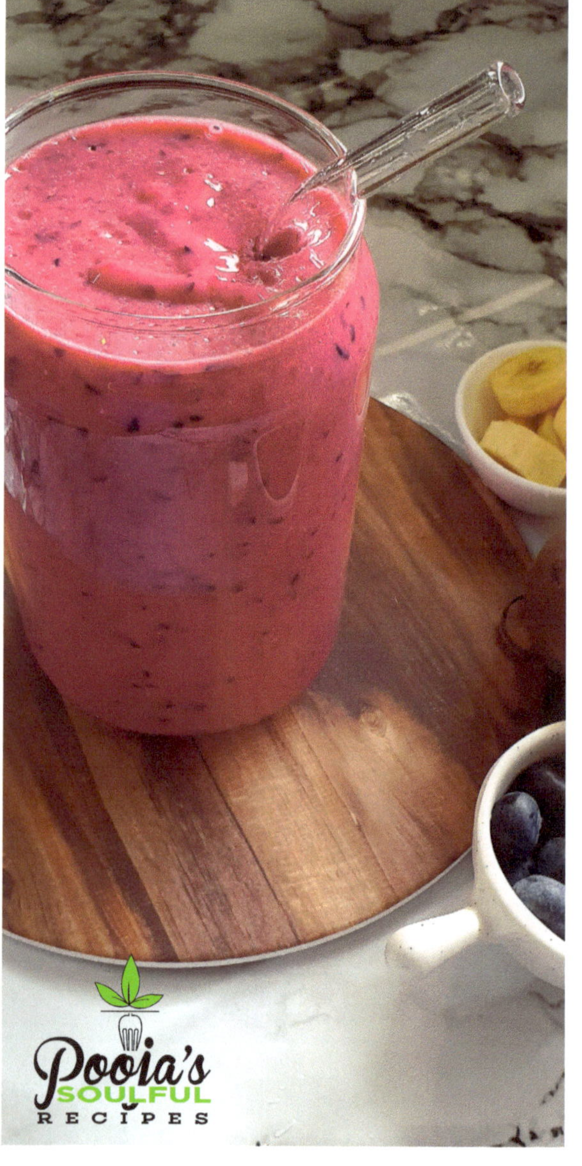

3. Taste and adjust flavors if desired by adding a sweetener if you prefer sweeter smoothies, or more lemon juice if you'd like some more tartness.

Notes -
- You can use any kinds of frozen berries for this smoothie.
- If you purchase beets with the greens still attached, you can save them and cook them like any other leafy greens.

Nutrition Information:
Serving Size:
1 smoothie

Amount Per Serving:
CALORIES: 239 | TOTAL FAT: 5g | SATURATED FAT: 2g | TRANS FAT: 0g | UNSATURATED FAT: 3g | CHOLESTEROL: 0mg | SODIUM: 393mg | CARBOHYDRATES: 45g | FIBER: 6g | SUGAR: 33g | PROTEIN: 7g

All nutritional information presented within this site are intended for informational purposes only. I am not a certified nutritionist and any nutritional information on www.seitanbeatsyourmeat.com should only be used as a general guideline. This information is provided as a courtesy and there is no guarantee that the information will be completely accurate. Even though I try to provide accurate nutritional information to the best of my ability, these figures should still be considered estimates.

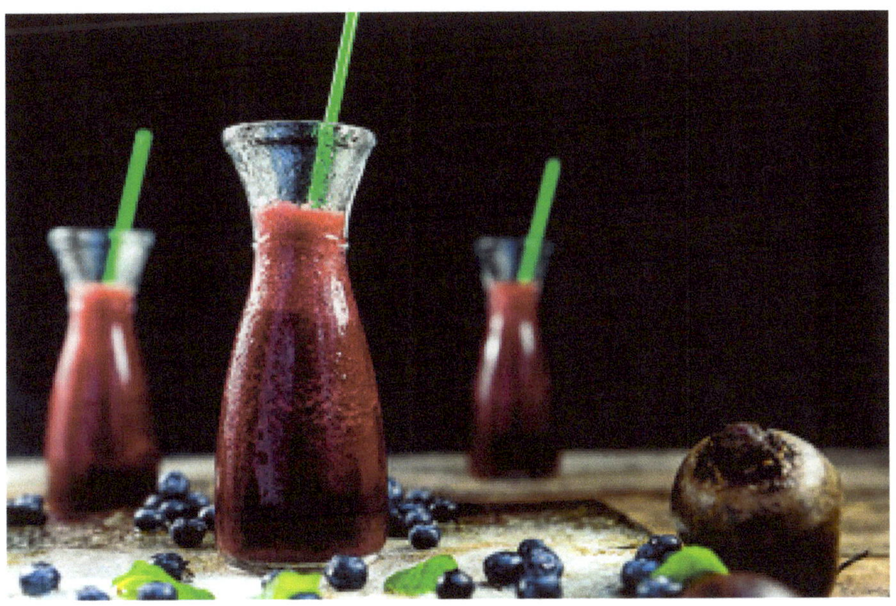

BEET ORANGE SMOOTHIE

Prep Time : 5 Minutes
Category : Smoothie
Method : Blender

This delicious vegan beet smoothie is easy to make with simple ingredients, high in protein and packed with nutrition.
Enjoy this bright and beautiful creamy blend any time you need a boost in energy.

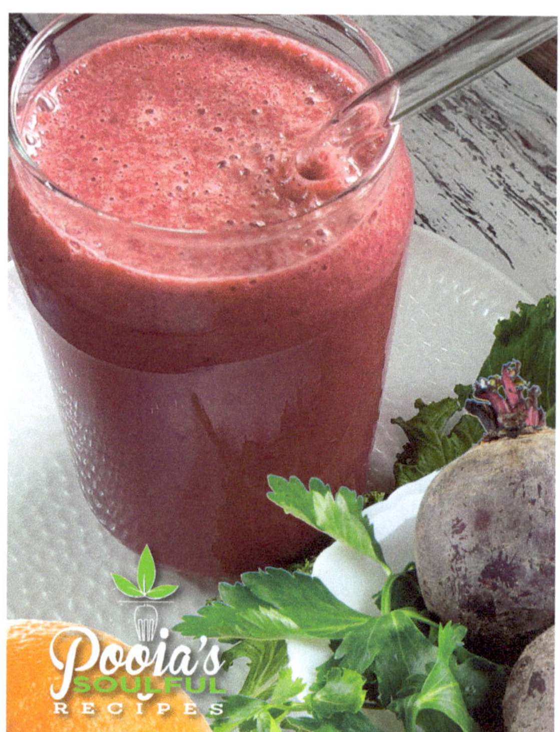

INGREDIENTS :
• 1 cup almond milk or plant-based milk of choice, plus more as needed to adjust consistency (250 ml)
• 1 small chopped beet, washed and root removed (100 g)
• 1 cup chopped and frozen zucchini rounds (100 g)
• 1 peeled and frozen navel orange (100 g)
• 1 cup or handful fresh spinach or kale (25 g)
• 1 scoop vegan vanilla protein powder (30 g)
• 1/2 a frozen banana, optional, for sweetening (or 3–4 small pitted dates)

INSTRUCTIONS :
1. Add the milk to a high-speed blender then add the rest of the ingredients.
2. Start blending on low then slowly increase speed, continuing to blend until it's completely smooth and creamy. You may need to stop a few times to mix it. Give it a bit longer than you think it needs to allow all the flavours to mix together and the beet to completely mix in. If needed, add a little additional milk to adjust the thickness to your liking.
3. Pour into a glass and enjoy.

INSTRUCTIONS :
Notes -
• This smoothie does have a hint of beet flavour to it so if you're not a big fan of beets, I'd suggest adding half a frozen banana for extra sweetness.
• To make this as a smoothie bowl, add the optional frozen banana, reduce the liquid slightly then blend on low until its thick and creamy, scoop into a bowl and enjoy with a spoon.

NUTRITION :
• Serving size: 1, Calories: 258, Fat: 4 g, Carbohydrates: 35 g, Fiber: 11 g, Protein: 25 g

MY DIET NOTES

MY DIET NOTES

MY DIET NOTES

MY DIET NOTES

MY DIET NOTES

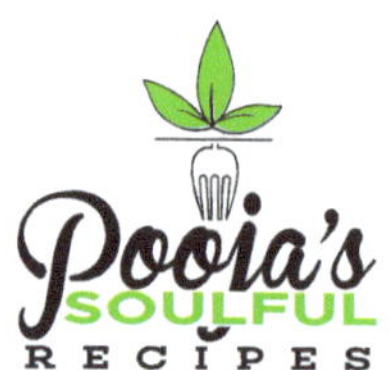

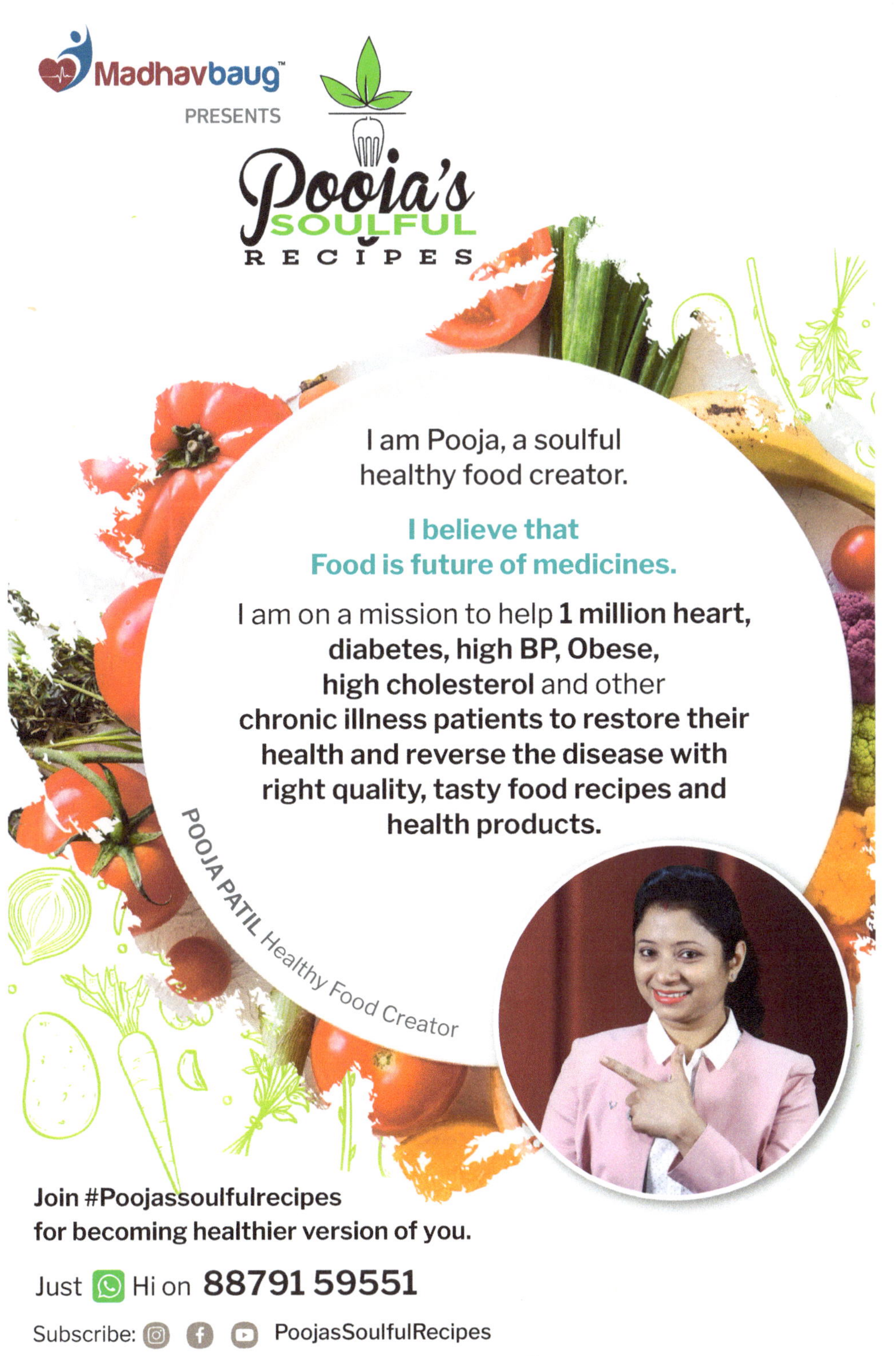

Madhavbaug™
PRESENTS
Pooja's
SOULFUL
R E C I P E S
I am Pooja, a soulful healthy food creator.
I believe that Food is future of medicines.
I am on a mission to help 1 million heart, diabetes, high BP, Obese, high cholesterol and other chronic illness patients to restore their health and reverse the disease with right quality, tasty food recipes and health products.
POOJA PATIL Healthy Food Creator
Join #Poojassoulfulrecipes for becoming healthier version of you.
Just Hi on 88791 59551
Subscribe: PoojasSoulfulRecipes
poojassoulfulrecipes@gmail.com
poojassoulfulrecipes.com

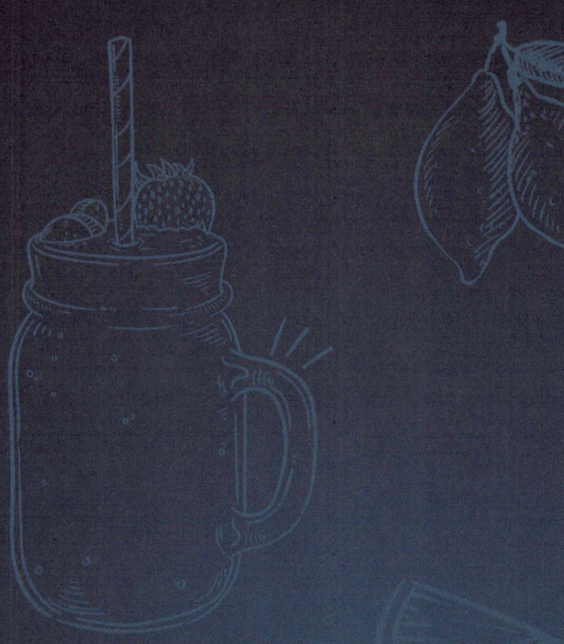
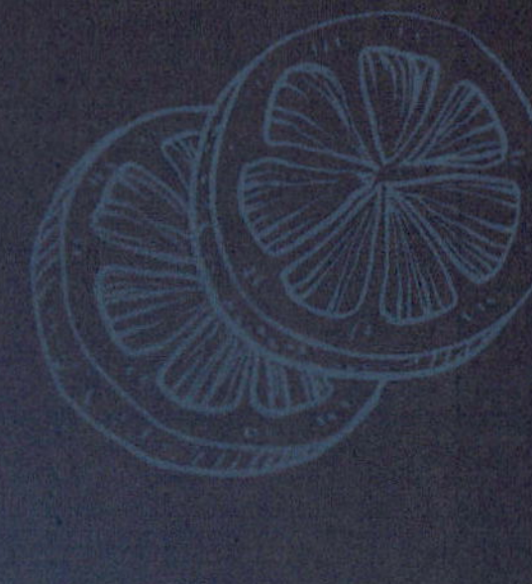
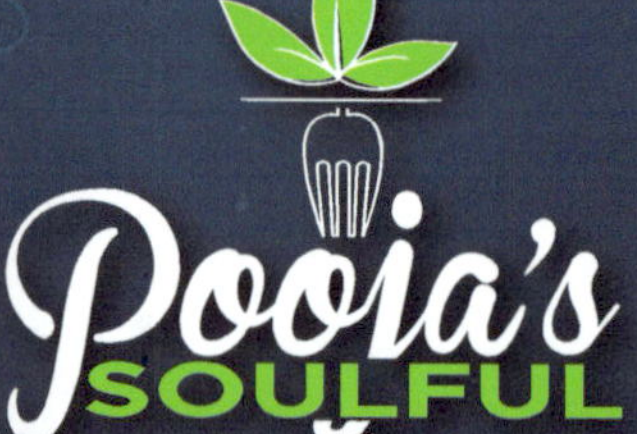

ISBN 979-8-3909-9260-9
9 798390 992609

MRP ₹229.00